# PRAYERS FOR CARE GIVERS

## Patti Normile

ST. ANTHONY
MESSENGER
PRESS

CINCINNATI, OHIO

*Nihil Obstat:* Rev. Lawrence Landini, O.F.M.
　　　　　　Rev. Robert J. Buschmiller

*Imprimi Potest:* Rev. John Bok, O.F.M.
　　　　　　Provincial

*Imprimatur:* +Carl K. Moeddel, V.G.
　　　　　　Archdiocese of Cincinnati
　　　　　　January 9, 1995

The *nihil obstat* and *imprimatur* are a declaration that a book is
considered to be free from doctrinal or moral error. It is not implied
that those who have granted the *nihil obstat* and *imprimatur* agree
with the contents, opinions or statements expressed.

Cover design by Don Nesbitt

Book design by Mary Alfieri

ISBN 0-86716-208-2

Published by St. Anthony Messenger Press
Printed in the U.S.A.

# Contents

*To the memory of*
Father Leonard Foley, O.F.M.,
*my dear friend and mentor,*
*who was a beloved spiritual caregiver*
*to unknown numbers of the faithful*
*and those who try to be faithful*

# Introduction:
# Caregivers and Caregiving

*Caregiver. I like that word, Lord. It says so much about who we are called to be in your Kingdom. Care indicates the deep regard we hold for others. Giver echoes the scriptural assurance that you love a cheerful giver. As giver I will strive to bestow on my patients your special gifts of faith, hope and love. I will attempt to empower them to use their own abilities and strengths. I will share with them the belief that your Holy Spirit is alive and well within them no matter what their physical condition.*

*Caregiver is who you are to me, Lord. May I give care to others in return.*

*So be it. So be it.*

"This isn't the way I wanted to grow old," Lucille murmurs. The sadness in her voice matches the melancholy in her eyes. "I'm not sure he even likes me anymore."

At eighty-four, the ninety-pound five-footer has cared for her six-foot-two, two hundred forty-pound husband since he suffered the stroke that changed their lives nine years ago. Her voice trembles with the pain and exhaustion of dealing with the daily needs of a once powerful, energetic man. This isn't the way either of them planned to grow old.

Lucille's distress brings to mind others I have met over the years, people who have had caregiving suddenly thrust upon them.

I remember my mom's tender care and strong resolve during my dad's dying months. I think of Peg's patient and loving care year in and year out for her daughter, Meg, who has Down's syndrome. I hear again Jody's anguished nighttime calls when her young husband lay dying with a bizarre disease diagnosed in only twelve other Americans. I recall Mary Jane's ability to keep happiness and humor alive as she cared for her husband, who finally lost all body movement to multiple sclerosis. He laughed the most when she let the pet gerbil she had bought scurry around the covers for a few moments.

I visualize the dozens of caregivers I have encountered while working in pastoral care in hospitals. I marvel at the courage and stamina of some caregivers. I ache at the resentment and anger of others. In most of them I have found a mixture of those qualities that rise and subside with the flow of daily caregiving.

Whatever their ages, their life-styles, their hopes, their abilities, all expected life to be different. They expected the aged to sleep quietly away some night. The young trusted that their children would be born strong and healthy, needing care for a few short years until they became self-sufficient. Those in the prime of life believed they and their loved ones were exempt from illness; accidents and injuries were events to read about in the newspapers or see on television. Extensive periods of caregiving were not included in their plans for the future.

I waited for Lucille to speak again. She took a deep breath and threw back her shoulders. With a gentle smile softening her face, she said, "Pray—just pray. It's the only way to get through each day."

"Just pray": She spoke a simple truth. Prayer is the way through troubled times. Prayer is not a magic wand to cure infirmities and illnesses. Prayer does not cause the healing pool of Bethesda to spring up in our backyards. Prayer may not alter the physical circumstances of our patients (though it sometimes does), but prayer can dramatically change *us* as we cope with life's challenges. As I consider those who meet the challenges of caregiving with the most grace, I realize each one is a person of prayer.

I promised Lucille that I would share with others her words about prayer as a source of strength for caregivers in the hope that the burdens of caregiving may be lightened. This book contains no miracle. The miracle is within you. Your untapped energies, your abilities, the faith still waiting in reserve enfold a miracle of kindness, perseverance and endurance yet to be revealed.

This book is intended to meet you "where you are." If your daily schedule has squeezed prayer into a congested corner of your life, it will encourage you to pray in new circumstances. If prayer has not been part of your caregiving, the book may inspire you to enter into caregiving prayer as a new experience. If prayer is your constant companion, perhaps you will find a new way to pray.

As you learn to trust the power of prayer you will find yourself moving to a new place in life. At times you may need to become like the performer on the flying trapeze: You will need to let go of some attitude, some stance in order to grasp a new hold. Prayer will enable you to look at anger and discover the underlying hurt. Prayer will allow you to forgive and find joy through reconciliation. Prayer can alleviate exhaustion with spiritual energy. Prayer will transform your thanksgiving into a gift to God.

## *One Family's Experience*

Let me tell you a story:

Jane's tennis game produced the first evidence of a physical problem. The former champion's body refused to respond with its usual agility and vigor. Initial physical examinations failed to reveal the source of the problem. Jane continued her daily activities, but progressive disabling symptoms crept in. Her husband, Bill, stood by her as they sought medical opinions. He was at her side when the diagnosis was given at the Mayo Clinic—ALS, incurable amyotrophic lateral sclerosis. Lou Gehrig, whose name the disease now bears, received the same diagnosis sitting in the same chair that Jane occupied. While Jane would receive no cure, she would receive much care. Bill became the center of her caring community. His organizational skills enabled him to assess Jane's needs, provide adequate care and alter plans as she deteriorated physically.

Bill learned to say, "I need you," to friends, neighbors and his employer. He moved his office into his home. Volunteer "Janie-sitters" were taught how to care for her and what emergency procedures to follow. Neighbors did the family's grocery-shopping and provided some meals. Friends played bridge with Jane long after she could hold cards or talk. (One blink of her eye meant, "Yes, that's the card I want to play." Two blinks meant, "No, try the next one.") A visitor to the family room, the center of activity, was quickly involved in a three-way conversation with Jane and Bill even though Jane could not speak. The one or two blink system, coupled with a relationship wherein Jane and Bill knew each other so well, almost made it seem that Jane herself was speaking when Bill became her spokesman. An abiding sense of peace and joyful life pervaded a home where death was inevitable.

Jane's death brought great sadness to the community. But those who had been part of her care team felt a healing sense of accomplishment in the care they had given their friend. Her family knew that they had loved her in the most caring way.

## *Challenge and Opportunity*

I tell you the story of Jane and Bill because caregiving is a challenging, demanding, exhausting, sometimes rewarding, often frustrating, frequently unchosen task. Observed from another perspective, it is opportunity. Caregiving provides opportunities to love, to alleviate pain, to enable healing, to grow in patience and wisdom and to experience life at intense moments.

Bill and Jane experienced the full gamut of struggle and loss through the months of Jane's illness. But they did manage to live with a sense of peace and joy during this period as together they discovered life's deeper meaning. The experience of caregiving can help both you and your patient to grow, to realize strengths, to discover life's meaning at a new level.

A newborn baby would survive only briefly without human care. We all react with anguish to an account of a baby wrapped in newspaper and found abandoned in an alley Dumpster. The thought of a tiny, helpless human being without someone to care for her, to hold and caress her, to feed and nurture her stabs our consciousness. Her predicament threatens our own sense of well-being. "What kind of world enables this to happen?" we ask.

Then we realize what a great need for love and care the child's mother must have. We know that she must not have been given adequate care in her life.

People must give and receive care throughout life in order to live as social creatures. Even the rugged old hermit of a western movie occasionally traipses into town for provisions or to have a painful tooth pulled. None of us exists without receiving care during our lives. Few of us live without caring for the physical, emotional or spiritual needs of others.

While caregiving is a fact of life, it can overwhelm you when the length and intensity of care required become more demanding. Caring for the sick or disabled can range in time from a brief period of tears in the night with a child who suffers from an earache to a lifetime of care for a severely disabled individual. In short-term caregiving, when your child stays home from school with a sore throat, the sickness is neither critical nor long-lasting. Caregiving can be a joy to your patient and to you, the caregiver. Special foods accompanied by quiet time together for reading or games create an atmosphere for renewed bonding between the two of you—patient and caregiver.

If your child is born with a chronic disability or develops a threatening disease, however, or when your loved one's aging or injury creates a need for months or years of caregiving, a different challenge exists. Caregiving means laying down your life, abandoning former activities to tend to your patient. Caregiving can mean helping someone deal with the anguish of severe or chronic pain or face the boredom of daily life without activity. Caregiving may offer the joy of participating in complete recovery from injury or illness, or it may entail sharing in the lifelong perseverance demanded by chronic disability.

## A Chosen or Accidental Role

Caregivers come in all ages, both genders, and any size and shape imaginable. Caregiving begins with a two-year-old who tells a sick mom, "I'll bring you a glass of water, Mommy." Caregiving extends to the couple married sixty-plus years who struggle on walker and cane to care for each other's needs through bouts of emphysema and crippling arthritis.

While all of us have some caregiver roles as spouses, parents, children and friends, intensified caregiving can enter our lives as chosen or accidental roles. If you chose to become a nurse, doctor, therapist, teacher, emergency technician or enter many other professions, you make a conscious decision to make caring for others a priority in your life. As a volunteer you may deliver meals to shut-ins, taxi patients to medical appointments, visit and read with them, tend to business matters, supply spiritual support. In these situations, your role as caregiver is chosen; it is learned through formal education, volunteer training, reading, hands-on experience and discussions with others.

Caregiving is professional when your income is derived from caregiving. Caregiving is relational when you and your patient are bonded by kinship, marriage or friendship. Caregiving is a volunteer endeavor when you choose to assist with patients' needs as a hospital, home or nursing home volunteer.

Whether professional, relative or volunteer, you as a caregiver are called to provide through your abilities and expertise for patients' needs.

Sometimes caregiver roles explode into your life without warning—accidentally, dictated by events in life over which you have no control or choice. As an accidental caregiver you are plunged into the unknown as the role is thrust upon you.

Real-life scenarios often alter life dramatically. John was an active, involved, soon-to-be-retired executive looking forward to travel and hobbies in his retirement years. Then his wife suffered a stroke that left her disabled. Their retirement years would be spent in unexpected confinement and routine. John became an accidental caregiver.

Bob and Thelma were not young when their first and only child, Margery, was born. She was the delight of their lives. Margery grew up and went off to college. That same year Bob suffered a heart attack that left him able to undertake only the most minimal activity. Thelma cared for him as Margery helped keep her mother's courage up.

Then one day Margery was riding her bike at college when a driver swerved off the road, struck her and kept on going. Margery was left with brain damage that impaired her sense of balance. Her mane of curly red hair bobs without control. She cannot walk. She is unable to sit without support. Thelma, angry, frightened, exhausted, in a brief time became an accidental caregiver to two people she dearly loves.

When you find yourself in an accidental caregiver role, you must scramble to gather information about your patient's needs. You determine whether the patient can best be cared for at home or in a nursing facility. Physical needs, financial and human resources all must be considered as you struggle to juggle the demands of everyday life with the responsibilities of caregiver. At the same time you are confronted with the emotions that the altered circumstances create in you and your patient.

You who are professional caregivers face similar strains in your careers, even though your entry into the caring profession is chosen. Karen became a hospice nurse after years of nursing in less intense circumstances. She recognized that her patience and love for those whose lives were nearing their earthly end was a unique gift. She decided to share this gift with those who had numbered tomorrows. Although Karen became a caregiver by choice, she still recognizes her need to deal with the loss of patient after patient.

Marcy, a single mom and nurse, became primary caregiver for Bernice during the final stages of Bernice's long struggle with cancer. Before her illness, Bernice had cared for Marcy's children. When Bernice's young adult sons were unable to care for their mother as her illness progressed, they remembered Marcy's compassion coupled with her nursing skills. The sons asked Marcy to take Bernice into her home to care for her.

Marcy gave Bernice her own bed. She accepted Bernice's rage and anger at her illness and approaching death. She provided a safe haven complete with the companionship of her children, for whom Bernice had cared. Marcy's whole family became caregivers by choice. During the time of caring for Bernice, they worked around the dynamics of an extra person in their home, one who required vast quantities of love, time and attention.

Role reversal creates a challenge as sons and daughters find themselves parenting their parents. The individuals who helped them walk and wiped their bottoms now require those services themselves. Children who remember receiving allowances from Mom and Dad now find themselves managing their parents' financial matters and perhaps their homes as well. In a topsy-turvy world where parent becomes child, the caregiver must strive to provide what is necessary without depriving the parent of roles he or she may still be capable of performing.

We must also face the undeniable truth that not all patients are nice people to be with. Penny's father had abandoned the family when she was in her early teens. The shame his drinking had caused lingered in her memory. The difficulties her mother experienced trying to provide food and shelter are still painful memories. Yet when her father was in need of medical care and attention, he appeared on Penny's doorstep for help. She cared for him until his death and even learned to love the old man, who still was not easy to like.

Some people have never made the top ten list of positive and pleasant personalities to begin with. Add the frustrations of being unable to care for themselves and the resulting anger, and you may have a monster under the bedsheets. Even those who get an *A* for amiability in normal situations may undergo a reverse metamorphosis from butterfly to worm when pain and disability afflict them. You may also have to contend with the chameleon personality—agreeable today, hostile tomorrow—as the stages of grieving an illness progress and regress.

Whether your role as caregiver is a chosen or an accidental responsibility, your ongoing duties will require immense resources of energy, organization, perseverance, patience and faith. As you become a fountain of life-giving care for your patients, you may find your own reservoirs of energy drying up. The flow of your patience may be blocked by anger or a sense of futility or hopelessness. The multitude of tasks may complicate the structure of your life. Your own state of health is an important consideration. Stress becomes a significant factor. Your perseverance may give way to despair. Renewal is essential.

Where can you go for renewal? Your caregiver role requires a system of friends, family and professionals for support with the physical, emotional, practical and spiritual issues that evolve from caregiving. A friend's offer to stay with a homebound patient will relieve you of your responsibilities for an hour or two. That time may seem like a week's vacation. A compassionate, nonjudgmental, listening ear can ease the built-up concern and pain inherent in caregiving. A meal prepared and delivered by a neighbor provides release from one of the day's tasks. Someone to field phone calls can free some of your caregiving time.

If you are not experiencing the strength of a

support system, you may need to learn to ask specifically for what you need. Boldness may be required because asking for assistance is an admission that you cannot do everything yourself. Most friends and family will be honored to hear the honest, heart-felt statement, "I need you." Ongoing caregiving places you face-to-face with the fact that you are not superhuman.

Most people wish to help you but are sometimes unsure about how to offer assistance. Would-be helpers may fear intruding into your private life. Facing serious medical situations may baffle or frighten some. You, the caregiver, or someone who knows the needs you and your patient face can best assess the situation and structure a system for effective support. Building a support system means more than rounding up a group of willing volunteers and establishing a schedule. Volunteers must be trained according to a patient's physical needs. Does he have difficulty swallowing? Can she walk or go up and down stairs? Does he have a catheter? What is the schedule for medications? What procedures should be followed should an emergency arise? Are any contagion procedures to be followed?

Those who enter the caregiver role with bombastic strength soon find themselves humbled. Joe used the skills he employed to run a factory to attempt to care for his invalid wife. Barking orders, controlling all of Helen's daily activities with rigid regimentation, he quickly discouraged others who wanted to be of assistance. Left with twenty-four hours a day of caregiving, he began to review the situation. Fortunately, he was open enough to discuss his dilemma with his pastor, who enabled him to look at a new model of organizing and working with other people.

Those who begin in fear and trepidation may encounter within themselves unexpected courage and confidence. Martha was a shy, unassuming woman whose life revolved mostly within the four walls of her home. When her husband, Harold, fell from a ladder, breaking both ankles and a wrist, she became the voice of his housepainting business. She parceled out his job commitments while seeing to Harold's recovery and rehabilitation. Her accomplishments enabled her to see herself in a new light as a capable businesswoman.

## *Going to the Source*

God, the Source of all life, all patience, all love, is our ultimate resource of strength and wisdom in caregiving. From ages past to the present time, prayer has been the channel for communicating with God. God's prayer line is open twenty-four hours a day. We can pray in any circumstances. Prayer takes no time yet can envelop all time. Saint Francis of Assisi advised:

> If you are upset for any reason whatever, you should immediately rise up to prayer, and you should remain in the presence of the Most High Father for as long as it takes him to restore you

to the joy of your salvation.

Times of caregiving can, indeed, create dramatic
upset. To experience such feelings is only human. To
remain in an upset state denies God's will for you. You
have the great resource of prayer during these times.

If caregiving makes you feel like the mythical
Atlas bearing the weight of the world on his
shoulders, count that as good. Atlas in his classic pose
has one knee on the ground; he is halfway on his
knees. Put both knees on the ground and you are in
one position for prayer.

## Using This Book

Scripture could not make more clear for us the role of
prayer, praise and thanksgiving in our lives. "Rejoice
always," Saint Paul writes, "pray without ceasing, give
thanks in all circumstances; for this is the will of God
in Christ Jesus for you" (1 Thessalonians 5:16-18).

The prayers that follow are intended as tinder to
light the fire of your own prayer. They are meant to
enable you to use the heat and energy of your anger
and frustration in positive, healing ways. They are
prayers to prime the pump of the wellspring of praise
and thanksgiving within you.

The prayers and thoughts of this book are inspired
by the experiences of individuals who lovingly care
for sick family members, friends and patients at
home, in hospitals and nursing homes. The hope is
that this book will make your work a bit easier, more

graced with praise and peace, more healing to patient and caregiver alike.

Its purpose is to provide prayers to keep the channel between you and God open and flowing with spiritual strength and energy. The prayers aim at illuminating the feelings about caregiving that rise within you. Hidden emotions like fear and anger may attack you from within. They can behave like an undiagnosed cancer, leaving you confused, weak and powerless. When feelings are acknowledged, named and accepted, they become more manageable. Emotions faced become part of the energy resources you need to continue your work of caregiving. Ongoing caregiving can dull the gentle senses of compassion, understanding and tenderness while leaving anger, frustration and resentment to run rampant. All feelings are valid; prayer helps to balance their effects in your life.

This book is not meant to be read cover to cover (although it can be). Glance at the Contents; flip through the prayers, seek a thought or word that appeals to you at this particular moment of your life. Are you tired, frustrated, angry, doubting, happy? Look for your feeling and pick a prayer that reflects your current attitude. As you finish with the prayers in the book, allow yourself to continue in prayer. These prayers are intended to jump-start your own communication with God, who longs to hear from you and is eager to speak to you in the quiet of your heart.

In your prayer, supply the names of the patients known to you and interchange feminine and masculine pronouns appropriately. Where a prayer trails off like this..., you may wish to continue with your own prayer.

The prayers of this book are *Emmanuel* prayers, "God is with us" prayers. Prayer does not beseech God to be with us. Prayer reminds us that God is always present; prayer reminds us to be with God. These prayers are yours to gather around you in a quiet corner of your life. These prayers are to fortify you in the most difficult moments of your day. These prayers are to help you to rejoice in the good that is present in any circumstance.

The prayers of this book are *now* prayers. Illness forces you to live in the present rather than the future. Pray for today and leave the future to God.

# Prayers to Greet the Day

The dawn of a new day may come with the optimism of the previous day's accomplishments. Sunrise may also bring heaviness of heart for caregivers. Unknown problems must be faced. Memories of yesterday's challenges may linger. A new day deserves a new chance. A day begun with prayer acknowledges that God is with you.

## Emmanuel

Emmanuel: God is with me today and every day.
Emmanuel: God is with me in my work.
Emmanuel: God is with me in my loneliness.
Emmanuel: God is with me in confusion.
Emmanuel: God is with me in the darkness.
Emmanuel: God is with me in my suffering.
Emmanuel: God is with me in my joy.
Emmanuel: God is with me in the everlasting.
Emmanuel....

## Good Morning, Lord

Gracious God, open my eyes to see you in this day.
Let me look for you in unexpected places and
people. When I fail to find you at first glance, give
me patience to seek further till I discover you in
every circumstance this day holds.

## Come, Holy Spirit

Come, Holy Spirit, fill me with your holy gifts
   today.
Send your strength to cover my weakness
      as I attend to today's duties.
Help me act with kindness and reverence for you
   and others.
Allow my words and actions to bring peace and
   healing.
May I harm no one with word or deed as I go my
   way.
Give me wisdom where I am ignorant.
Encourage me in my doubt.
Deliver me from temptations.
Comfort me in sad moments.
Hear my prayer, Holy Spirit.
Fill me with your light
      that I may grow in holiness and love.

## One Day at a Time

One day at a time—just live one day at a time. I've known the wisdom of that admonition for many years. I try to live that way, Lord, but in this time of difficulty I find I'm living my "one day at a time" in the wrong era.

The day I attempt to live may be a day in the future as I wonder what our lives will be like a year or two from now.

The day I live may be in the past as I remember good times and easier circumstances.

One day at a time can only be in the present. Once again I will praise you for one day—*today*—just as it is. I will live today with a sense of joy in knowing that you, Lord, are with me through each exquisite moment. One day at a time is *now*!

## Smile

I will smile today, Lord.
Much is happening that may not seem to merit
    smiles,
        but I will smile today.
I will smile because a gentle smile reduces stress.
I will smile because to frown would not change
    anything.
I will smile because my smile may light up
    someone else's life.
I will smile and someone may mirror that smile
    back to me,
        and I do need a smile today.
I will smile as witness to the world
        that nothing can separate me from the joy
        of having you in my life.

## A Gift

Today, like every day, is your gift to me, Lord. I will
endeavor to give it back to you by caring for others
and myself. Guide my actions. Guard my mouth.
Give me wisdom to carry on today.

# Prayers of the Senses

The five senses—sight, hearing, taste, smell, and touch—are sources of human learning. These senses also provide links to other humans. Aging and illness can compromise these senses. As they diminish, a sense of isolation creeps into the patient's life. Food neither tastes nor smells as good as it once did. Loss of hearing often leaves one feeling abandoned in the midst of a conversation. Visual impairment immerses one in a fog of unknowing. Aging skin can either become hyper-sensitive or suffer a diminished sensitivity to touch.

As caregiver, you will become aware of the need to recognize and stimulate these senses to add vitality to the life of your patient. You may describe a sunset to one with failing vision. You may speak louder, slower, more distinctly for the hearing-impaired individual. You may search for foods that trigger the patient's appetite. You may splash a bit of after-shave or cologne on a freshly washed body. And you can touch the skin in gestures of love and concern for the patient.

## Tenderness

Lord, the loneliness and isolation of the elderly
swept over me in a wave of sadness today. For
some, years—even decades—have passed since
they have experienced the intimacy of a hug, a kiss,
a shared moment with a loved one. Without those
tender touches in their lives, they have retreated
into their protective shells like threatened turtles.
One grouched at another who touched her chair in
passing. Another grumbled when a visitor stopped
to chat. Still another grasped her purse for fear a
passer-by would snatch it.

Few things are worse to lose than intimacy, Lord,
unless it is knowing our need for intimacy. I
probably cannot change what years have carved
into hearts hardened by life's lost tenderness, but I
thank you for making me aware of the need for the
intimacy of touch and shared tender moments. I
will seek to give and receive tenderness today.

## Another Day

I really don't want to be here today, Lord.
The sounds of sickness haunt me—
    moans and groans and an occasional outcry.
The smells of illness invade my being
    and linger when all is fresh and clean again.
I dread the sight of ailing, failing bodies—
    some bloated, some with skin draped over
      bones
    as if someone had sucked the muscle out—
the feel of skin so lifeless and so cold
    I wonder for a moment if life still pulses
    beneath its pallor.

But I'm not here alone.
You are with me in twofold fashion:
    in each patient I tend
    and within me as well.
I really don't want to be here today, Lord,
    but together we can make it through the day.

## In a Foreign Land

Dear Lord, she seems an alien in a foreign land.
Life-support systems sustain her in an atmosphere
    now too rare to uphold her life.
Nourishment drips into a body that once relished
    lasagna, roast chicken and vegetables *al dente.*
It hurts to see her in this jungle of tubes and beeps.
    She belongs in her garden of tulips and
      birdsong.
Perhaps we are all aliens in this land—
    just waiting for our return trip home.


## The Oldest Form of Healing

You touched the leper, Lord,
    and he was made clean.
You touched eyes with spittle,
    and the blind could see.
Before medicines and surgeries,
    healing came through touch.
Let my touch heal hearts and hurts.
Let my touch say,
    "You are fearfully, wonderfully made."

## Fragrances

Lord, if I recall the fragrance of summer's roses,
    of spring showers when life bursts forth from
      the earth,
if I remember the smell of powdered babies'
    bottoms,
    of suntan lotion on my children's skin,
if I recreate in my mind the pungency of spices and
    herbs
    wafting from a kitchen in full swing,
then just perhaps I can tolerate the smells of
    sickness
    that do not vanish.
Some, like alcohol, are not obnoxious, it's true.
    But other smells attack my nose with a
      vengeance.
I cannot hide from them.
    They penetrate my every breath
    and linger when all is pristine again.
Lilacs, bacon sizzling, coffee in the pot, Aqua Velva,
    pizza, honeysuckle, pine forests—
Lord, fill the memory of my senses with fragrance.

## Awakened Senses

Have you intensified my senses, Lord,
   to compensate for hers that weaken?
I seem to hear with the ears of a fox
   small sounds unnoted before—
      the rustle of a sheet (Is she comfortable?),
      the sound of a cough (Is she choking? I'll
         check.),
      a murmur that's more like a whimper (Is
         the pain coming back?),
      a breath that sounds raspy (What does it
         mean?).
Then sometimes the silence deafens my ears.
Life is for sound.
Thank you, Lord, for the sounds that silence my
   fears.

Out! Out!

Why is it, Lord, that no breath can clear my head of
   it?
No fresh air drives it out.
I feel as if the lining of my mind is coated
       with the taint of urine, excrement and other
          body smells.
I've washed and talcked.
The bed is changed.
The disinfectant smell seems almost as bad,
       but still I fear that visitors may detect
       an odor that is not pure.
I fear it will offend a nose
       and indicate I have not done my job—
       that somehow I've neglected him.
I'm getting somewhat like the lady who with
   obsession
       declared, "Out, out damned spot!"
Instead I say, "Out, out damned smell!
   I banish you forever from my head!"

## Changing Sights

On a recent yesterday she looked young.
> Today she is old.
Only yesterday it seems I saw her strong.
> Today she is feeble.
Just a yesterday ago she was vibrant.
> Today life seeps away.
Did my sight deceive me, Lord?
Did she really change so rapidly?
I wonder how you see her, Lord,—
> young and strong or old and feeble?
What my eyes see is only external.
What you see is eternal.
Lend me your eyes, Lord.
Please lend me your eyes.

## Searching

You remember, Lord,
>we used to look eye-to-eye as we talked—he
>and I.
We searched each other's minds through the
>windows of our eyes
>>to seek the deeper meaning of our words.
Now my eyes search his face;
>his eyes are veiled in unknowing.
I search for signs of recognition,
>for his mouth to form a word.
I look for signs that life goes on,
>a shallow breath in, a soft breath out—
I look, I search....

## Skin

O Lord,
You wrapped our humanness in skin at our
    creation.
I spend so much time caring for skin—
    cleansing it,
    watching for signs of sores,
    observing its transparency,
    testing its warmth,
    softening it with creams,
    anointing it with oils.
Though it first appears that you gave us skin
    to hold our body-stuff together,
    I think you provided skin for touching.
A caress of a brow says,
    "I long to take your pain away."
The enfolding of a hand means,
    "I am with you."
The stroking of an arm reminds us of strength
    that surpasses muscle tone.
A back-rub seeks to bring relief and relaxation.
Thank you, Lord, for skin for touching.

# Prayers of the Emotions

E motions are integral to our humanity. Yet we
sometimes struggle with how to handle our
emotions. Rampant emotions seem to grasp
you by the arm and drag you through torments of fear
or anguish. Emotions can also sweep you up in a tidal
wave of joy. The wise person knows that feelings are
neither right nor wrong; they simply *are*.

Emotions can be easily denied. You smile and say,
"Oh, no, I'm not angry," while you seethe inside. "It's
OK," you bravely state when your inner self writhes in
pain. You sometimes feel inhibited about expressing
unbridled joy.

These prayers attempt to acknowledge that
emotions simply *are*. They are present in your life.
They are powerful in your relationships. Without
them you would be an emotional corpse. Security
always lies in expressing your emotions to God. That
can be the first step in sharing them with others.

## Hypocrite

I confess, Lord, that I felt like a hypocrite when he told me how patient I am with him. I know the grinding impatience that sometimes screams in me. My mind spills out a thousand silent reprimands: "Why can't you try?" "If only you would...." "A little effort on your part would...." "Oh, my God, not again!"

Patience? Of course! He sees your patience in me. Your Spirit quells my angry words and halts my thoughts before they break upon the world of sound. Your Spirit speaks within me, reminding me that hard times end and kindness is worthy of one who follows you.

To you, Lord, I can release all the anger and frustration that wells within me. The space released is free to be filled with that fruit of your Spirit—patience.

## Losing It

I feel as though I'm losing my soft side, Lord; my
gentleness is vanishing. My responses sound
harsh, monosyllabic. My mouth feels as hard and
tense as the words that burst from it all too often.

Could it be that the core of my being has been
tempered—hardened—by the heat of each day's
challenge? Have the fires of anxiety that burn in me
transformed my soft side into rigidity? I would
rather be a gentler self—warm and willing, flexible
and free.

How can I become gentle once again? I may need to
reenter the fire and surrender my control to you.
Your word tells us that fire also burns the dross
away, leaving purified metal.

I have been afraid of being hurt if I am soft. The
greater danger may be that I will hurt others if I am
hard-tempered and sharp of tongue. Recreate me
as a gentle self, Lord.

## Angry!

I'm angry! There, I've admitted it. I'm angry
because I watch the game she plays. She is
recovering quite well. When I visit for her therapy,
she seems positive and "up."

Yet if a family member or friend comes or calls, a
new person emerges. Her normal voice becomes
weak as she murmurs a frail, "Hello." Her
shoulders sag. Her face, where moments earlier
courage had shown, settles into sad resolve. "I'm
OK, I guess," she tells her caller in a small voice
plagued with doubt.

I really fume inside when I see her manipulate with
feigned weakness those who offer their support.
Does she know she does this, Lord? Does this
projected image of herself as weak and frail delay
her recovery? I don't know the answers.

Guide me, Lord, to love her through this time. If I
am to bring awareness to the situation, let me do so
in gentle confrontation guided by your Spirit.

## Families

Where is her family, Lord? No one has come to visit
for such a long time. She looks toward the door of
her room many times through the day. "Has
anyone called?" she asks with hope. Her question
fills me with sadness and anger. What can I say
except, "Not that I know of," and extinguish her
hope. They are all so busy, or so they say. She is
not busy; she has all day. One brief visit, one call
would give her thoughts to live with for days to
come. Her family makes me angry. They make me
sad.

## Gentle Yet Strong

Gentleness must never be confused with being
    weak.
Great strength exists in gentleness.
Gentle wind powers the sailboat over the waters.
Gentle encouragement calls forth undreamed-of
    potential.
Gentle persuasion married to perseverance
    contains the might of steel.
Lord, keep me gentle. Keep me strong.

Joy!

*Joie de vivre*—the joy of life!
It somehow sounds better in French,
    but, though it means many things to many
        people,
    to me it always means *you*.
You, Lord, are the joy of my life!

Joy is a living thing, Lord.
    Because it lives, it requires nurturing.
Today you kept joy alive in a myriad of mini-ways—
    Sarah's smile,
    Jack's "Thanks, hon,"
    Bertha's holding my hand,
    Henry's apology....

You were present in each person and each tiny
    event.
Thank you for being the joy of my life.

## Two of Me

Two houses, two yards, two families, two jobs—
  Since he is sick there seems to be
  double of everything for me to care for.
I really want to help, Lord,
  but why didn't you make me twins?


## Not Yet

I've tried, Good Lord, I've tried,
  but I cannot give up my anger yet.
My love for him will not permit me to let my anger
  go.
I want him well again. He is so special, so precious!
In a way I feel my anger is all that holds me
  together.
Without it I might collapse
  into a mass of uncontrollable pain and sorrow.
Yes, Lord, I'm angry with you, too.
You healed so many, many people—young and old.
  Why not him? Why....

# Prayers for Times of Doubt and Discouragement

I n the quiet of the night, amid the confusion of changing circumstances, in the light of a new diagnosis, doubt and discouragement raise dragon-like heads. You can succumb to them or you can challenge and overcome them. Each time you overcome the demons of doubt and discouragement, you build within yourself confidence that you can carry on in your caregiving role.

What If...

What if I'm not with him, Lord,
    when you come to call him home?
What if I can't hold his hand to steady him
      as he crosses the chasm of death from life to
        life?
What if he cries out and I don't hear his call?
What if words hang in the rattlings of his throat
    and I'm not there to hear?
What if...?
    What if...?
    What if...?

You'll be there, of course, even if I am not,
    doing all I could and infinitely more.
Thank you, God, for releasing me
    from the burdens of "What if...?"

## Visiting Nurse

Visiting nurse—it sounds like one who drops by
  for a cup of tea and social chat.
Sometimes I wish my job could be more like that.
  Today it's a blind mom and her retarded son.
  How long can they continue on their own?
I don't want to play your role.
  I'm not God to decide who stays and who goes.
Then on to visit three women
  crippled by arthritis, bent with pain.
  One has admitted that crawling is easier than
   walking.
If they could only live together.
  Each could lift the other up—
  at least in spirit.
  But, no, it cannot be.

Maybe I'll just sit down
  and have that cup of tea.

## An Answer

How will it be, Lord,
> when this long battle for his life is over?
I know I'm supposed to live just one day at a time
> yet sometimes a real fear wells within me.
Maybe I'll always remember him as he is now—
> frail, sometimes angry, sometimes stony
>> silent.
Will the frustration and anger of today blot out
> memories of
>> pony rides and picnics,
>> Christmas trees and sled rides,
>> singing songs as we drove along,
>> surprise gifts and electrician lessons?
I seem to hear your answer, Lord.
You ask me, "Did Good Friday erase the memory
> of Christmas or of the Resurrection?"

## Decisions

My life seems threatened by an avalanche of
   decisions, Lord.
   By rights these choices don't even seem mine
      to make.
My mom and dad always encouraged me to make
   my own choices.
   Now I am forced to make some major ones for
      them.
Where can Dad be cared for? Can Mom bear to be
   away from him?
To sell or not to sell the house
   that has been their home for more than fifty
      years—
If we don't, where will the money come from to
   care for them?
If we do, will the loss of that old place
   take a final toll on them?
I ask them what they think will be best.
The answer is a tear-filled eye, a shoulder shrug
   or "You know what's best."
I have the feeling that no answer will be totally
   right.
Help me, Lord, to find solutions that are the best.

## Weary

I'm so tired, Lord, so very, very tired.
My feet ache.
My legs feel weak.
My head throbs.
I am so tired.
I try my best to do all the everyday tasks my life
   demands
      and care for her special needs, too,
      but I'm wearing down.
What am I to do? I must keep on giving but
      I have little left to share....

I'm beginning to understand:
      To give we must also receive.
Others have offered help—
      an errand run,
      an hour of time,
      a listening ear—
      but I have been too proud, too self-sufficient.
"Thanks so much," I say, "but I can manage.
      Everything's just fine."
I'm so tired because
      I've deprived others of the privilege of giving.

Forgive me, Lord, for my proud selfishness.
The next time I'll respond,

"That would be great. I could use some help!"
Better still, I'll honor a friend
    and ask for what I need.

## Doubting

> *No distrust made [Abraham] waver concerning*
> *the promise of God, but he grew strong in his faith*
> *as he gave glory to God, being fully convinced that*
> *God was able to do what he had promised.*
> *—Romans 4:20-21*

O Lord, I long to be like old Abraham. Today I
discovered that I still am not. I know your promise
is to bring us to peace and everlasting life, yet
sometimes I doubt. Oh, I don't doubt your
presence, Lord. I doubt my own ability to follow
you.

Once again I will place doubts and questions in
your care. I'll stop right now to give you the glory.
You will strengthen my faith and fulfill your
promises.

Glory, praise and honor be to you, my loving God!

## Rainy Season

This long illness seems like a perpetual rainy season. Each day one expects the sun to shine, but the sky remains thick and foreboding. The sun of promise seems shrouded forever. The storm of pain pounds against the roof of my heart.

How do I deal with rainy days that affect the climate of my life? Perhaps I can cope with them as I do with rainy weather—a cup of tea, a good book, a heart-to-heart talk with a special friend, a task attacked and accomplished, a time to pray. All these provide safe haven when stormy days rage outside. They may be just what I need to face the clouds of doubt that mist my view of tomorrow.

## Above the Fog

The fog of that vacation morning has taught me much about living with the uncertainty of illness. Looking down toward the water it was visibility zero. Only the sound of the incoming tide announced the presence of the invisible water. The shrouded morning was punctuated by the bleat of the fog horn that directed the fishing boats to the sea. But when I looked up from the third floor window, I saw blue sky and sunshine layered on the fog's surface like icing on a cake.

In the midst of caring for the sick, I sometimes feel like I am in a fog that blankets my view of the future. Sounds may direct me—a patient's request, a doctor's orders, a family's question, a chaplain's prayer—but the outcome is still unseeable.

Memory of the fog reminds me that above all the unknowns, beyond the unseen, you are ever present, Lord. The warmth and light of your love are always present beyond the fog.

## Self-Doubt

Self-doubt sits on my shoulder like a small,
irritating imp. This imp whispers in my ear, "You
blew it, stupid."

In my other ear I hear you speaking, Lord: "Good
work. You did the best you could today. Tomorrow
will be even better."

Away with you, imp of self-doubt who sits on my
shoulder! I brush you away like flakes of dandruff.


## Help!

Help me, Lord! So many need so much!
I feel I am gathering eggs in a basket far too small.
Each lonesome, ailing soul I visit becomes
    another precious, fragile sphere of life
    to bear to you in prayer.
I need your help to balance my basket of care.
I want no one to fall unloved.
Show me how to bring into these lives
    the warmth of love to nurture their rebirth of
        hope.

## Endless

Lord, I do believe a forest has been destroyed to provide paper for forms to chronicle his illness. Applications, receipts, statements, instructions, documentation, medication listings, apparatus bills and government interrogations—is there no end to the paperwork?

Then to find the information! Here is 1963's complete financial record—household, taxes, medical, auto battery guarantee and dog license— all tied up with string so tidily. But where is this year's data? Where can I begin? Where do I request duplicate information?

Paper, paper everywhere! How I shrink from this task! Save me, Lord, from death by paperwork!

## Burnout

Someone dared to diagnose my dis-ease today,
   Lord.
I didn't even know I ailed.
Yet as I think about the symptoms,
I guess I've caught a giant case of burnout.

Frustration has replaced satisfaction.
Anger squelches my peace of heart.
Weariness robs my energy.
Tension rigs my body taut as a set trap.
Smiles refuse to soften my face.
I find no time to listen.
I'm flying on automatic pilot from one task to the
   next.
The fever of responsibility has consumed me.

I must be healed.
You are my Creator, Lord.
I offer you my time, my will, my total self.
Heal me. Recreate me, Lord.

## Drought

Lord, I feel as if I'm caught in the throes of
summer's drought. My reservoir of strength and
energy is dry and barren. Long hours, little rest and
little thanks have left me weary and frustrated. I'm
a caregiver with little left to give.

I guess I'd better give *myself* some care. I'll begin
by giving myself permission to take time off. I'll ask
for help. I'll laugh and play a bit. I'll allow time for
your love to flow into my reservoir of faith and hope
and love.

I confess I've been playing God, thinking I can do
all, be all. But only you are all in all.

## Keeping On

Lord, I have one thing to say,
       just one thing to pray:
Help me to keep on keeping on.

## Meddlesome

Does his family come to visit? or do they come to
criticize? Each time they're here, the gripes I hear!

I listen with hopes of satisfying them. Then I
realize that will never be. Criticism is their way of
communicating their dissatisfaction with life. No
change will bring content. I'll do my best, Lord.
And they, poor souls, will have to live with
themselves and their discontent.

## Facing Death

Dear Lord, we called his friends and relatives to tell
them how critical he was. Few came; there were
few cards, few calls. But when he died, they all
were there. How he would have loved to have seen
them a few weeks earlier! Dying is very difficult to
face. Sometimes facing death is easier.

## Prayer for Death

She looked at me with pleading eyes, Lord, then asked softly, "Is it wrong for me to pray for him to die?" We talked about God, the Creator, the Author of life, recalling that God is also the Author of *eternal* life.

We remembered that in the Garden of Gethsemane you asked your Father if the cup of death could pass you by. Yet you yielded that request to God's own will.

We considered her husband's long struggle with illness, his vanished vigor, the pain that racks him night and day, his own wish to be free of the burden of living. "What do you wish for him when you pray for his death?" I asked.

"To be free of pain. There's no hope of recovery."

"You want him free...."

"That's it! I want him free to live eternally. I guess I just want to say that I am ready for God's will to be done. I pray for death so that he may have life."

Praise you, Lord, for your victory, which transforms the darkness of death into the hope of life!

## Prayer at Death

It's over, Lord. The suffering and anguish have ended.
At his death I'm overwhelmed with gratitude for
  his life!

Lord, thank you for the goodness of his life,
  for the scars from which that goodness grew.

Thank you for the wisdom of his life.
Praise you for the adversity that produced such
  wisdom.

Thank you for his faithfulness.
Praise you for the questioning that strengthened
  his faith.

Thank you for his love so lavishly bestowed.
Praise you for the yearnings that spawned love.

Thank you for the peace his presence brought.
Praise you for the restlessness that made his peace
  such a gift.

Thank you for his generosity in giving of himself.
Praise you for the sacrifices that created his
  generous spirit.

Thank you for his relentless hope.
Praise you for death, which bears the hope of
  everlasting life.

# Praying Through the Stages of Grief

The stages of grief associated with the dying process also apply to grieving the losses injury or illness imposes. Elisabeth Kübler-Ross identified and described the stages in *On Death and Dying*: denial, anger, bargaining, depression and acceptance. Even when illness is not life-threatening, loss looms for the patient and often for you, the caregiver. Time away from work may cause concern for job security. Inability to perform one's everyday roles as parent, spouse, child can attack self-esteem. Separation from peers may create loneliness. Apprehension about full recovery or disfigurement may be cause for grieving.

As caregiver, you are faced with a double dose in the grieving process. You must acknowledge your own sense of loss as well as your patient's grief. The closer the relationship between you and your patient, the more complex the link between your grieving stages may be.

To complicate matters further, stages of grieving are not predictable and progressive. Both you and your patient may bound from one stage to another with little warning. A new symptom may plummet one who had reached a healthy stage of acceptance right back into anger. The more that you and your patient are able to discuss with openness the feelings engendered by the illness or injury, the greater the possibility will be for handling your grief in a healthy manner.

## Sojourner

I am a fellow traveler with him
    as he journeys the road of his illness.
I cannot know precisely how he feels—
    his fears, his hopes, his pains, his triumphs.
Yet I am willing to explore with him
    the experiences of this illness.  How can we
        bypass the roadblock of a new complication?
Where will a detour lead us as we try a new
    treatment?
Can we slow down and be at peace on a bumpy
    stretch of recovery?
How will we survive the potholes of anger, despair
    and frustration?
Who will be in the driver's seat?

Help me, Lord, to remember that this is his life
    and his illness we are traveling through.
I am a sojourner, traveling this journey with my
    friend.

# *Denial*

*Denial reflects the mind's refusal to comprehend at the moment the reality of serious illness or injury. Denial is not a negative unless it persists for an extensive period. A short period of denial gives your patient and you time to gather the emotional and spiritual resources to face the facts and cope with them.*

## This Can't Be!

Oh, God, this can't be happening. He looks so healthy and, until the diagnosis, he was a happy man. We always believed that a seed of life lives in every blossom. How can a seed of terrible illness lurk within the bloom of his life?

## Dancing With Denial

Denial holds me close...
    all this anguish will go away quite soon.
Then I spin away to truth:
    The doctor's words were clear.
Denial draws me near again where I'm snuggled
    and secure.
    I pull from denial's grasp and push it far from
      me.
Denial reels me close again.
    Truth beckons one more time.

When will this dance be over, Lord?

# *Anger*

*Anger surfaces when the veil of denial begins to drop.
The injustice of illness or injury rages in your soul and
boils to the surface, often spilling over to anyone present.
Anger contains abundant energy to put to constructive
use if you can harness it.*

## Too Good

He's much too good for this, my God!
He cares for others and himself as you yourself
   would do.
His whole life is a portrait of kindness in action.
The poor always get his gifts of time and money,
   too.
The bereaved he visits long after others do.
Unfairness sends him off to seek justice.
Help me to understand!
He's much too good for this, my God!

## Erupting

My anger dulls my senses, Lord.
My mind can only cry out, "Why?"
I cannot seem to do a thing.
My rage consumes my will to act.
I want to hit, to cry, to scream
at the injustice of it all.

I trust that after the volcano of my rage—
the smoke, the fire, the flow—
when the eruption of my anger slows,
you will guide me through its fiery paths
and lead me to new life beyond my raging, angry
    state.

Why?

Why? Why? Why?
Why must things be as they are?
Give me a new question, Lord.
I see there is no answer to my angry *why*?
Give me *what*: What actions shall I take?
    What can I do to move on with life?
Give me *who*: Who has gone this way before?
    Who can help me see my way?
Give me *how*: How will I take care of just today?
    How can I turn my attitude around?

Thank you for new questions, Lord.
    I'll work with them instead of asking why.

## In Anger

Lord,
sometimes I get angry, really mad,
and I say or do things
that I later regret.
Then I apologize for the cutting remark,
the cruel accusation.
But apologies aren't always enough.
There may be no way to undo the harm.
Help me to accept my temper as a reality.
Help me to control it and direct it
into constructive channels.
Help me to harness my anger
so that it will move me to work
to relieve the oppression of the poor,
the needless slaughter around the globe,
the destruction of earth's beauties.
Above all, help me to learn restraint.
For a moment's hesitation
can mean
preventing a lifetime of regret.

*(Leonard Foley, O.F.M.)*

# Bargaining

*Bargaining is the "I've got a deal for you, God" stage where promises and propositions are offered in exchange for good health and recovery.*

## Let's Make a Deal

My practical nature longs to strike a deal. I begin to negotiate a mental bargain. "Lord, if you will..., I will...." I'd do anything to have my way, to have her well again!

As these thoughts congregate in my mind, I realize how futile they are. You have already gifted me with everything. Your gifts of life, of love, of eternal life, of yourself are all mine already. For all my bargaining there is nothing greater you could give than what you have already showered upon me.

I will give to you, Lord, in return for your abundant gifts. I will try to give myself, my will, my trust, my love and my loved one. No bargains, no deals. Please accept my little gift, Lord. Thank you for your great gifts.

## Bargaining

I know I haven't always lived the way I should have, Lord. I've made a billion excuses for my shortcomings and sins. Is that why things are in the mess they are right now?

Forgive me, Lord. I'll try to live your way. Can I have another chance, Lord? Just once more, please?

You say you haven't punished me, that my sins bear self-inflicted punishment. These circumstances stem from living in the world where life and death grapple in each human life.

I don't need to bargain with you, Lord. You have overpowered death with resurrection's power.

# *Depression*

*Depression creeps in when denial departs, anger abates
and bargaining does not produce instant health of body,
mind and spirit. The actuality of injury or illness finally
reaches the mind, which must now wrestle with reality.*

## Depression

I need your help, Lord, when caring for her. She is
depressed. A part of me wants to say, "Buck up, old
gal! This too shall pass!" Of course, that is neither
wise nor professional, but I confess it still lingers
on my lips.

Depression is a bit like quicksand. If you thrash in
its grasp, it may pull you ever deeper. I must move
gently with her, supporting her until she finds firm
emotional ground. Then she can step beyond the
hold of depression's dark doubts to acceptance of
her situation and herself.

## Fear

Thank you, Lord, for showing me that I am a bit afraid of his depression. I guess I fear it is some contagious, virulent disease that I don't want to catch! I don't want its debilitating effects to rob me of life's energy as it has taken his away.

With your help, Lord, I will review and renew my view of depression as a phase of grieving one's illness. Depression is a time when the spirit seems to slumber. You are always present through this time, empowering the person to move nearer to you.

Give me courage and patience to stand by him through this time.

# Acceptance

*Acceptance brings peace of mind. The reality of the physical condition, the required treatment necessary and the circumstances prescribed for patient and caregiver are accepted as part of life. Acceptance is not synonymous with giving up. It is more like letting go of nonessentials in life. Acceptance lives peaceably with reality.*

## Approaching Death

The approach of death is like a crack in the chalice of life. No way remains to plug the leak as the elixir of life flows out. Yet just as certain as the reality that life is flowing away from this earthly existence is the realization that life is flowing into the eternal. Our choices are to cling to what we will inevitably lose or to pour it out freely. I choose to give freely, Lord.

Better Half

You made us one, Lord,
    and now my better half is leaving me.
A slow departure to be sure, but inevitable
    and not so very far away.
She grows so weak.

She also calls me her better half.
That must mean that between us
    we are more than one whole couple.
That can only be because you are in our marriage—
Two better halves plus one better whole.

What will I be when she is gone?
A lesser half?
No, I don't think so.
Her spirit self will stay with me
and you will rest in both of us
    always and forever.
I feel your comfort in believing that.
I'm a bit more ready for the inevitable.

## Prayer of Abandonment

Father,
I abandon myself into your hands;
    do with me what you will.
Whatever you may do, I thank you;
    I am ready for all, I accept all.
Let only your will be done in me,
    and in all your creatures—
I wish no more than this, O Lord.

Into your hands I commend my soul;
I offer it to you with all the love of my heart,
for I love you, Lord,
and so need to give myself,
to surrender myself into your hands without
    reserve,
and with boundless confidence,
for you are my Father.

*(Brother Charles of Jesus)*

## 'Terminal'

Someone used the word *terminal* last week, Lord. I
have known deep inside that she is nearing the end
of this life. But *terminal* sounded so harsh. Yet
when I look at the word I remember that the word
has another sense, that a terminal is a place where
we change planes, trains or buses to journey to
another destination. She is approaching the
connection point to eternal life. Give me the
strength to help with her needs at this crossroad
between this life and the next.

## On the Shore

My Lord, as her life ebbs, it seems as if she is being
carried away by the strong tow of the outgoing tide.
I am forced to stand on the shore and watch her
slip into the deep unknown. I am so thankful that
you are the Lord who walked on the water. You will
be with her.

# Bits and Pieces

Among these prayers, which reflect a bit of one person's emotions in dealing with disability and a piece of another's heart in facing difficulty, you may find a fragment of your own hope springing from despair, your own strength growing from weakness, your own faith spawned from doubt.

## For the Sick

Lord, your life on earth was filled with concern for the sick. Have compassion now on all who share your pain. Give them healing of mind and body; restore their strength and spirit.

May they be comforted by the knowledge that we are praying for them, and find peace in a sense of your presence. May they know that in a special way they are united with your suffering. May they contribute to the welfare of the whole people of God by associating themselves freely with your passion and death for the salvation of the world.

Bless those who take care of the sick. In their own time of need, may they receive a hundredfold the blessings they have given.

*(Leonard Foley, O.F.M.)*

## Hide and Seek

I've lost her, Lord;
She has gone away.
Oh, she appears to be here still—
    in body, that is,
But the person who dwelled within that familiar
  form
    seems to be playing hide and seek.
Sometimes she hides behind
    an invisible veil of silence.
Other times she darts into an unknown world
    of other people, places, times and things.
What hurts the most is when she cannot find me
    in this game of hide and seek,
    and I'm right here beside her,
    waiting to be recognized, wanting to join in.
When she hides, I long to call out,
    "All-ee, all-ee in come free,"
    and have her come from her hiding place
    to be with me again.

## Swinging and Clinging

How she clings to life, Lord.
Like the trapeze artist hanging from the bar,
    she careens from the security of this life
    toward the safe haven of the next.
Just when it seems her life is spent
    and she will fly to you,
    she grasps the day with renewed energy.
Your waiting arms,
    outstretched to lift her to eternal life,
    remain empty.
She fears falling into the deep abyss.
She has always loved you, Lord,
    yet she fears her sin is greater than your love.
She fears that you will drop her
    when you touch her sinfulness.
Send your Spirit to reassure her, Lord,
    that you are not only the arms that await
    but also the eternal net of mercy
    awaiting all who might fall.

## Walking Backward

Lord of our journey,
I feel I'm walking backward in time,
caring for the mother who gave birth to me,
who brought me fresh from you.
She encouraged my initial steps across to Dad
and led me in prayerful steps to you.

Now the process is reversed.
I walk with her,
supporting unsure steps that falter.

In prayer we return to you, our Father.
Thanks and praise to you, Lord God,
for this round-trip ticket
and the blessing of such a treasured travel-mate.

## A Puzzlement

Oh, Lord, his life is a puzzlement! For a dozen years he has slept baby-style, curled as in his mother's womb, the haven he left nearly a century ago. Unlike a babe, he does not wake to cry and churn the air with thrusting feet and fists. He sleeps.

We feed him a soft puree of nourishment. He is bathed and clothed. He sleeps.

His family comes hundreds of miles to visit. "Hi, Dad. We're here. We love you, Dad. Can you wake up?" He sleeps.

"Dad, we want you to know we are all OK. We will be just fine if you want to go to be with Mom. She has been gone three years now. It's OK. We will be just fine. We love you, Dad." He sleeps.

I look for meaning in his life that appears so lifeless. He is loved. Love brings life where it does not seem apparent. Perhaps his silent spirit already rests with you, and only we who look for outward signs of life are puzzled by his lengthy lingering in this world.

## Images

Lord, today I'd like to be an artist painting
images—not on canvas but in the mind: images of
wholeness created with broad brush strokes of
hope and promise. If I can capture the images of
health hidden in today's pain and illness and paint
them in my patients' minds, tomorrow may find
those images come to life.

## Whole Being

As I care for him, Lord, help me to remember that
I care for an entire person, not just body parts that
ache and pain. As I tend to his dressings and bathe
his body, help me to care for the entire human
person wrapped within. His irritable personality is
linked to an unhealed wound of spirit. Fear causes
him to strike out with angry words. Long years of
loneliness cause him to hide from friendship
offered. Please use me, Lord, to help mend the
fragments of his life.

## Mindful of the Moment

You put a phrase into my mind, Lord: "Be mindful of the moment." That thought has drifted through my mind all day. It affected everything I did. The traffic light that seems eternal some days gave me time to pray. The tense and troubled woman in the elevator seemed relieved by the few words we shared. I've tried to be mindful of each and every moment I have spent with patients, to dedicate that time to you.

The result has been astonishing, Lord, and I give thanks to you. It seems this day burgeoned with extra grace-filled time. I might have consumed the day without awareness if you had not cautioned me, "Be mindful of the moment."

## Knowing When

Knowing when is such a challenge, Lord,
    when to confront,
    when to let go,
    when to do,
    when not to do,
    when to agree,
    when to stand firm,
    when to question,
    when to affirm.

Asking for the gift of knowing when
    is just another way of asking for your wisdom,
      Lord.
You know my need.
Please hear my prayer.

## Sick Versus Sickness

He is not a *sick person,* Lord;
    he is a *person with a sickness.*
Help me to remember that.
A person with a sickness
    possesses health as well as sickness.
To call one a sick person
    indicates that only sickness exists.
Sickness and health wrestle with one another
    in those who struggle with sickness.
I choose an alliance with health
    when I see him as a person with a sickness.


## Nosey

"I won't leave this life," she protests. "I'm too
nosey. I want to know what is going on!"

Pain wracks her body, yet she clings to life. Being
nosey is an interesting reason for living in pain,
when letting go might gain heaven. That vantage
point could satisfy her hunger to know what's
going on.

## Listening

Thank you, Lord, for ears. Please connect mine to my heart. This heart-connection will enable me truly to listen to the feelings others share with me. With heart-listening I may even hear words that are not spoken, those too shy to venture into the world of sound. When two souls meet in heart-listening, each becomes stronger through the union.

## An Honor

When I was young, I never ever thought I could return all the good my parents did for me—encouraging me when I was discouraged; loving me when I was unlovable; believing in me when I didn't know who I was. Now I *know* I can't repay them in equal portion. But thank you, Lord, for the opportunity to do some things for them that they can no longer accomplish on their own. Thank you for the wonderful privilege of giving a little in return for their great kindness and love....

## Living Is Changing

Lord, you have made me an observer of life. As I
watch my patients' lives, I recognize life-style
changes. Some changes are chosen; others
imposed. Some changes require letting go; others
mean taking responsibility.

However alterations in life come, they remind me
that being alive means always changing. Change
can be arduous. Change is also my opportunity for
new growth, new life.

Keep me ever aware, Lord, that change happens
not just to others but to me. What change do you
ask of me today? What am I to surrender? What
responsibility shall I accept?

Keep me truly alive through changes in my life,
Lord.

## Forgive Me, Lord

I really do believe in that little phrase,
"I'd rather be right than have my own way."
But today, I forgot about it and insisted on my way.
Mine was not the right way.
Mine was not your way, Lord.
Mine was the stubborn way.
Mine was the selfish way.
My way hurt others.
My way made others angry.
I ask your forgiveness, Lord.
I also need courage to ask forgiveness
        of those whom my willfulness has injured.
I am sorry. I am so sorry. Forgive me, Lord.

# Night Prayers

At day's end you may experience a variety of feelings—gratitude for opportunities to serve, frustration at unresolved issues of the day, heartache for what seems unchangeable, pain inflicted by angry patients, exhaustion from the day's work, a mind full of thoughts about tomorrow. Sleep brings restoration. The more unencumbered you are as sleep approaches, the more renewing the night's rest will be. Night prayers allow you to transfer to God's care what you cannot care for through the night.

## An Evening Prayer

Lord, as I lie down to sleep tonight
    I trust you with the burdens
    that I have gathered up today.
Many cares were lifted
    by joys sprinkled through the hours,
but some concerns for those for whom I care
    linger in my thoughts.
Help me to tuck them
    securely in my heart
to free my mind
    for rest and peace tonight.
My heart will not forget those
    whose problems do not fade
but will love them till the dawn
    without the worry of my mind,
which seeks solutions to problems
    that lie in your hands alone.

## Another Day

We made it through another day, Lord—you and I.
I could not have come the way alone.
Others try, I know,
    and think they can do all on their own.
But even they are guided by you,
    unknown to them, in myriad ways.

Thank you, Lord, for shepherding all your flock
    along our way today.

# Just for Me Prayers

You are very special to God and to others. Use these prayers—"just to lift your spirit prayers," "just to give you joy prayers," "just to get to know you prayers"—to talk to God about you.

## Make Me a Gentle Breeze

*(A reflection on 1 Kings 19:9-12)*

Lord, make me a gentle breeze.
Let me stroke the heads of little ones.
Send me across the gnarled faces of the old.

Lord, make me a gentle breeze.
Allow me to dry the tears on the cheeks of the
    bereft.
Let me skip over the teardrops
        on cheeks of those whose cups run over with
            joy.

Lord, make me a gentle breeze.
Let me move among your people
        caress them, hold them, love them.

Lord, make me a gentle breeze.
May I stir the spiritual waters of those who are still.
Keep me gentle lest I overwhelm the still more
    gentle.

Lord, make me a gentle breeze.
Let me rest assured
        in the Source of my strength lest I become a
            wind.

Lord, make me a gentle breeze.

Use my passing to bear your Spirit where you will
    to lift hopes, scatter doubts and bear despair
    away.

Lord, make me a gentle breeze.
Give me a prayer to whisper as I flow.
Let me murmur praise for everything.

Lord, make me a gentle breeze.

## Happy Birthday!

I'd like to sing "Happy Birthday" to me today, Lord.
It's really not my birthday, but I have the desire to
sing that little tune to let you know that I am so
happy that you gave me life to live and to share
with others.

Thank you, Lord, for giving me life.

## Who Am I?

Lord, I am who I am—but who am I?
It sounds like a riddle, Lord—the riddle of myself.
Every once in a while I say something and ponder,
 "Where did that come from?"
Or I act and wonder,
 "Did I do that?"
Sometimes I think and say and do
 what doesn't seem to be me
 and it's good and I'm thankful.
Sometimes I think and say and do
 what doesn't seem to be me
 and it is not so good.
Then I think,
 "I'd like to discard what isn't genuinely me
 and keep what is wholly and truly me."
I'd like to seek and keep
 only the truth that is me—
 not someone else or who I hope to be—
 just simply, wholly me.
The truth seems to be
 that there's good and there's bad within me.
The *ultimate* truth seems to be
 that I am one whom you love
  with the good and the not-so-good still in me.

# Prayers of Praise and Thanksgiving

Faithful pray-ers say that if we pray enough, all prayer becomes praise and thanksgiving. The more you take your needs, your pain, your frustration to God, the more clearly you will see the bounty that God has already placed in your life. From that realization arise praise and thanksgiving.

## Rejoice and Give Thanks

Rejoice in the Lord always; again I will say, Rejoice. Let your gentleness be known to everyone. The Lord is near. Do not worry about anything, but in everything by prayer and supplication with thanksgiving let your requests be made known to God. And the peace of God, which surpasses all understanding, will guard your hearts and your minds in Christ Jesus. *(Philippians 4:4-7)*

## Little Things

O, Lord, you know how I've always loved small things—miniature horses, doll houses, Lilliputian-sized books, a vase big enough for a single violet blossom.... Now I've learned to love other small things, tiny joys: the hint of smile that says he is comfortable for a while, the whisper of a kiss on my ear as I lean close to hear the faint sound that forms a word, the squeeze from a hand once strong and capable, now frail and letting go of life.

Thank you, Lord, for tiny joys.

## Joy!

Joy! That's what I long to give to you today, Lord,
joy!
Joy is one of the really good gifts I can share with
you
because you give it first to me.

I felt a sense of joy when I first awoke this morning.
Joy drifted in on an early sunbeam.
Joy wafted in the fragrance from my cup of
coffee.
Joy pelted me in the warmth of my morning
shower.

Joy is more than happiness that comes and goes.
Joy comes when every cell of my being is energized
by your Spirit.
Thank you for the joy of living in your Spirit.

Thank you, Lord, for this precious gift to give to
everyone I care for today.

## Memories

O, patient Lord,
When days bog down in endless tasks—
    counting pills and changing beds—
I thank you for thoughts of silly things
    that tickle me within
    and plant a smile on lips ready to complain.

I remember steeplechases with Mom
    across the bushes from back porch to garage
    when we were grown women.

I recall an escapade in water ballet with my
   daughter
    as hotel guests watched bemused
    (and, I think, a bit envious
    of our unbridled and unself-conscious fun).
If anyone saw resemblance to a sounding whale,
    they kept it to themselves
    although opinions would not have spoiled our
     joy.

I picture snow angels of past years
    imprinted in the snows of time and memory—
    some large, some very small.

And I plan in my busy mind
    a particularly foolish folly for very, very soon.

And now back to counting pills and changing yet
another bed.

## A Bouquet of Thanks

I'd like to gather all the thanks she gave to me and
present them to you, Lord, like a huge bouquet of
roses. She could not stop saying, "Thank you for all
you've done for me!" I replied, "You're welcome."
She is truly one who is welcome, welcomed into the
land of those who are grateful of heart. I did not do
much for her; I just listened. I tried to listen as I
believe you listen, Lord—without judgment, with
love and concern. Please accept this bouquet of
thanks, Lord.

## Gifts

Thank you, God of gifts, for the gifts you shower upon me. Perhaps I don't think about them for fear of becoming proud. Now I realize that they are all from you and to ignore them would be ungrateful on my part.

I often take for granted my patience and my tolerance. Thank you for giving me the will to wait when others fidget and fret.

My problem-solving skills save me from many a dilemma. Thank you for a mind that sees beyond the quandary to discover an answer.

Thank you, God of gifts, for....

## Stepping Stones

Praise your wisdom, dear Lord, for allowing the difficult, the hard things in my life. At first they seem to be obstacles: immovable, firmly planted in my way. When I realize I cannot move them, I accept them—and find they are stepping stones.

Without these hard things that become stepping stones, I might never venture across the swift-moving stream of life. I might be swept away by powerful currents or stay where I began, on the barren shore of self. With you to steady my steps, I can cross to the fruitful side of the stream. A bounty of peace, love, hope, joy, kindness, goodness awaits me there.

If I hesitate midstream, fearful of the next long step, afraid of plunging into the stream or, worse still, tempted to stay and bathe in quiet, still waters that may become stagnant, I know you will allow another stepping stone—hard, firm, immovable— to ease my crossing over to you.

Praise your wisdom, Lord, for allowing the difficult, the hard things in my life.

Thanks for...

Thank you, gracious Lord,
> for the softness of a baby's skin,
> for aged eyes that twinkle still,
> for fresh baked bread and ice-cold milk,
> for sunsets and sunrises, too,
> for the whippoorwill's call,
> for a friend's smile,
> for your Spirit alive in me,
> for....

I give you thanks and praise, most giving, gracious
Lord.

# Prayer of the Imagination

Often you do not have the luxury of time, place or space for a sit-down or kneel-down prayer time with God. Such busy times are frequently when you need prayer the most. God has given you the gift of imagination, which can provide the place and space for prayer. You must still carve time from busyness to create this prayer of the imagination in your mind. After it is recorded there, it requires little time to bring it forth anytime during your day when you need to pray.

To create your imaginary prayer space, take some sit-down time to program your imagination. You may first wish to record the following prayer of the imagination on a cassette tape. Replay the tape, following its suggestions as you sit in a quiet, peaceful place free of disturbances. Allow ten to fifteen minutes for this initial experience.

Speak slowly as you record. You may want to play some peaceful, instrumental music in the background as you read.

Sit in a comfortable position in a straight chair, feet flat on the floor, hands relaxed in your lap. An erect back and closed eyes complete the body's preparation for prayer.

Allow all tension to flow from your body....

Breathe out tension....

Breathe in peace....

Breathe out anxiety....

Breathe in peace....

Breathe out anger....

Breathe in peace....

Search for places of tension in your body....

Relax your shoulders....

Slacken your jaw....

Feel the weight of your hands at rest in your lap....

Using God's wondrous gift of imagination, you are going to create a place for prayer, a place to which you can return at any time in the future. This place will be exclusively yours. This place of prayer will be made sacred and holy by the Lord's presence in it. Once it is etched upon your memory it can be reentered instantly as circumstances in your life demand.

You are walking in a meadow, knee-deep in lush green grass. The softness of the grass invites you to remove your shoes. You feel the cool blades cushion each step as they wrap around your toes and cradle your feet. As you walk, you slow your pace to observe your surroundings.

A gentle breeze causes the grasses to sway like slender dancers moving in harmony to an unheard rhythm. You feel a longing to slow your own life to that tempo, to be in harmony with the rhythms of nature.

The sun is pleasantly warm, like the touch of God's grace brushing your face. As you walk, you discover a small stream sparkling as it meanders through the grassy meadow. Shiny gray stones and darting fish can be seen through the crystal-clear water. Several large stones link to create a pathway across the babbling water. You may cross on them or walk through the refreshing waters.

Wildflowers of every imaginable color dot the soft grasses. Birds swing, singing, through the gentle breeze. Pine trees loom in the distance. You smell their fragrance wafting over the meadow.

You continue walking slowly. You try to enfold every beauty the day has to offer. You draw near the woods. As you walk into the towering presence of the pines, you feel the coolness of their sheltering shadows. The sun mottles the pine needles strewn on the forest floor. The mystery of the woods beckons you. You walk deeper into the trees. You move in quiet wonder at the glory of the tall trunks reaching toward the light. The trunks are now enormous. The trees tower above you. The light is dim and subdued.

Just as you consider turning back because of the growing darkness of the woods, a clearing appears. Ringed by pines that have stood for decades in this place, it is wreathed in soft, filtered sunlight. A fallen tree rests near a large rock in the center of the clearing. You hear an unspoken invitation: "Stop and rest awhile." You may sit on the rock or on the fallen tree.

You have never felt so totally alone—yet you are not lonely at all. You sense a powerful presence near you. A figure enters the clearing. A man approaches. His clothing is simple, his feet bare like yours. You experience no fear. From the man's very being an aura of love exudes.

You realize that you are in the presence of the Lord Jesus Christ. You drop from your sitting place to kneel before him, but he takes your arms, encouraging you to return to your seat. He settles down beside you. Though you have many questions you have always wanted to ask him, words seem unnecessary. Your body feels energized by his power and strength coupled with his gentleness. You experience a sense of well-being that surpasses all heights of health, happiness and peace.

His eyes look into yours—into your very being, into your spirit. In their look is all the love and forgiveness and healing you have ever longed for and infinitely more. You respond with wordless love and praise. Now he speaks in a voice rich with the resonance of eternity. Pause for a few minutes and listen to what he says to you.

As he finishes speaking, he invites you to share with him what is in your heart. You speak....

He listens, absorbing every word. His smile reassures you that your message has been received with love. You remain, content to be silent with him.

As he stands to depart, he tells you that this special

place will always exist in your heart. You can return at any time and he will meet you here. He enfolds you in a tender embrace, then slips silently back into the deep woods. The clearing glows with the lingering light of Jesus' presence.

Before you depart, take another long look at your surroundings to engrave this place on your imagination. Slowly open your eyes.

Remember that you can always return to this special place of prayer. It is engraved on your imagination and on your heart.

# Journaling

J ournaling chronicles the day-to-day emotions and realities of caregiving. A pen or pencil, a blank page of paper and a few minutes of the day can be used to create an invaluable map of your own emotional and spiritual journey on the road of caregiving. Journaling provides a way to unload burdens acquired in the ongoing care of another person or persons. Committed to paper, a fear, a frustration, a victory or an accomplishment assumes concrete reality. You can celebrate your victories. You can face your fears and rediscover hope.

You may protest that you have no time to maintain a journal. But a journal does not have to be a literary masterpiece. A few words jotted down will remind you of your feelings at a particular time. As you read them later, you will see the pattern of your journey. The journal provides tangible evidence of how you survived difficult challenges. Journal notes remind you of joyful moments and hold the promise that they will come again.

The journal is a place to record a word of thanks or

praise from your patient or another person. You can return to it when you need to affirm the value of yourself and your work.

Add a poem, a prayer, a proverb, even a cartoon that lifts your spirits to your journal to create your own caregiver's gospel—the Good News that God is present in caregiving.

The following questions offer a guide for reviewing your day. Reflect on them as you write in your journal:

- What did I allow myself to learn about me?
- What did I allow myself to learn about patients and their families?
- What did I allow myself to learn about sickness and health?
- What did I allow myself to learn about my theology?
- Where is God in this?

(Notice the key word *allow*. Each of us has many opportunities for learning in any given day. We need to give ourselves *permission* to learn and to be changed by those experiences. The challenge is to see how to learn and grow in negative experiences as well as positive ones.)[1]

Journaling can be a valuable way of caring for yourself, the caregiver.

[1] Patti Normile, from *Visiting the Sick: A Guide for Parish Ministers* (Cincinnati, Ohio: St. Anthony Messenger Press, 1992), p. 108.

# When Prayer Doesn't Seem to Work

You pray for a loved one to recover and her condition deteriorates. You pray for healing and death slips in instead. You pray for strength and feel overwhelmed by your weakness. When you reach a place in life where prayer does not seem to be working, you may want to reexamine your concept of prayer.

Prayer is not a wish list directed at God, complete with deadline for delivery. Prayer is not a way to manipulate God through pleadings and petitions to arrange the universe according to our way—even if our way seems totally good and right.

Prayer is a path to God. Along that path you carry everything to God—your praise and thanksgiving, your hopes and needs, your joy and suffering. You leave them with God as your gifts of love and trust. In return you receive the ability to accomplish what you thought impossible, to love someone you thought intolerable, to continue when you believe you cannot endure. Through prayer you will someday be showered with the realization that God is present to you through the joyful and agonizing moments of life. Prayer always works because God is always with you.